MedicalCenter.com

The Key Facts on Attention Deficit Hyperactivity Disorder (ADHD)

Everything You Need to Know About ADHD

-Usable Medical Information for the Patient-

By Patrick W. Nee

www.MedicalCenter.com

Published by:

MedicalCenter.com

96 Walter Street/ Suite 200

Boston, MA 02131, USA

Tel: 617-354-7722

www.MedicalCenter.com

manager@medicalcenter.com

Table of Contents

Chapter 1: Introduction

What is attention deficit hyperactivity disorder?

Attention deficit hyperactivity disorder (ADHD) is one of the most common childhood disorders and can continue through adolescence and adulthood. Symptoms include difficulty staying focused and paying attention, difficulty controlling behavior, and hyperactivity (over-activity).

ADHD has three subtypes:

- Predominantly hyperactive-impulsive
    - Most symptoms (six or more) are in the hyperactivity-impulsivity categories.
    - Fewer than six symptoms of inattention are present, although inattention may still be present to some degree.
- Predominantly inattentive
    - The majority of symptoms (six or more) are in the inattention category and fewer than six symptoms of hyperactivity-impulsivity are present, although hyperactivity-impulsivity may still be present to some degree.
    - Children with this subtype are less likely to act out or have difficulties getting along with

other children. They may sit quietly, but they are not paying attention to what they are doing. Therefore, the child may be overlooked, and parents and teachers may not notice that he or she has ADHD.

- <u>Combined hyperactive-impulsive and inattentive</u>
    - Six or more symptoms of inattention and six or more symptoms of hyperactivity-impulsivity are present.
    - Most children have the combined type of ADHD.

Treatments can relieve many of the disorder's symptoms, but there is no cure. With treatment, most people with ADHD can be successful in school and lead productive lives. Researchers are developing more effective treatments and interventions, and using new tools such as brain imaging, to better understand ADHD and to find more effective ways to treat and prevent it.

Chapter 2: Symptoms of ADHD in Children

What are the symptoms of ADHD in children?

Inattention, hyperactivity, and impulsivity are the key behaviors of ADHD. It is normal for all children to be inattentive, hyperactive, or impulsive sometimes, but for children with ADHD, these behaviors are more severe and occur more often. To be diagnosed with the disorder, a child must have symptoms for 6 or more months and to a degree that is greater than other children of the same age.

Children who have symptoms of <u>inattention</u> may:

- Be easily distracted, miss details, forget things, and frequently switch from one activity to another
- Have difficulty focusing on one thing
- Become bored with a task after only a few minutes, unless they are doing something enjoyable
- Have difficulty focusing attention on organizing and completing a task or learning something new
- Have trouble completing or turning in homework assignments, often losing things (e.g., pencils, toys, assignments) needed to complete tasks or activities
- Not seem to listen when spoken to

- Daydream, become easily confused, and move slowly
- Have difficulty processing information as quickly and accurately as others
- Struggle to follow instructions.

Children who have symptoms of <u>hyperactivity</u> may:

- Fidget and squirm in their seats
- Talk nonstop
- Dash around, touching or playing with anything and everything in sight
- Have trouble sitting still during dinner, school, and story time
- Be constantly in motion
- Have difficulty doing quiet tasks or activities.

Children who have symptoms of <u>impulsivity</u> may:

- Be very impatient
- Blurt out inappropriate comments, show their emotions without restraint, and act without regard for consequences
- Have difficulty waiting for things they want or waiting their turns in games
- Often interrupt conversations or others' activities.

ADHD Can Be Mistaken for Other Problems

Parents and teachers can miss the fact that children with symptoms of inattention have the disorder because they are often quiet and less likely to act out. They may sit quietly, seeming to work, but they are often not paying attention to what they are doing. They may get along well with other children, compared with those with the other subtypes, who tend to have social problems.

But children with the inattentive kind of ADHD are not the only ones whose disorders can be missed. For example, adults may think that children with the hyperactive and impulsive subtypes just have emotional or disciplinary problems.

Chapter 3: Causes of ADHD

What causes ADHD?

Scientists are not sure what causes ADHD, although many studies suggest that genes play a large role. Like many other illnesses, ADHD probably results from a combination of factors. In addition to genetics, researchers are looking at possible environmental factors, and are studying how brain injuries, nutrition, and the social environment might contribute to ADHD.

Genes

Inherited from our parents, genes are the "blueprints" for who we are. Results from several international studies of twins show that ADHD often runs in families. Researchers are looking at several genes that may make people more likely to develop the disorder. Knowing the genes involved may one day help researchers prevent the disorder before symptoms develop. Learning about specific genes could also lead to better treatments.

Children with ADHD who carry a particular version of a certain gene have thinner brain tissue in the areas of the brain associated with attention. NIMH research showed that the difference was not permanent, however, and as children with this gene grew up, the brain developed to a normal level of thickness. Their ADHD symptoms also improved.

Environmental factors

Studies suggest a potential link between cigarette smoking and alcohol use during pregnancy and ADHD in children. In addition, preschoolers who are exposed to high levels of lead, which can sometimes be found in plumbing fixtures or paint in old buildings, may have a higher risk of developing ADHD.

Brain injuries

Children who have suffered a brain injury may show some behaviors similar to those of ADHD. However, only a small percentage of children with ADHD have suffered a traumatic brain injury.

Sugar

The idea that refined sugar causes ADHD or makes symptoms worse is popular, but more research discounts this theory than supports it. In one study, researchers gave children foods containing either sugar or a sugar substitute every other day. The children who received sugar showed no different behavior or learning capabilities than those who received the sugar substitute.

Another study in which children were given higher than average amounts of sugar or sugar substitutes showed similar results. In another study, children who were considered sugar-sensitive by their mothers were given the sugar substitute aspartame, also known as Nutrasweet. Although *all* the children got aspartame, half their mothers were told their children were given sugar, and the other half were told their children were given aspartame. The mothers who *thought* their children had gotten sugar rated them as more hyperactive than the other children and were more critical of their behavior, compared to mothers who thought their children received aspartame.

Food additives

Recent British research indicates a possible link between consumption of certain food additives like artificial colors or preservatives, and an increase in activity. Research is under way to confirm the findings and to learn more about how food additives may affect hyperactivity.

Chapter 4: Diagnosis of ADHD

How is ADHD diagnosed?

Children mature at different rates and have different personalities, temperaments, and energy levels. Most children get distracted, act impulsively, and struggle to concentrate at one time or another. Sometimes, these normal factors may be mistaken for ADHD. ADHD symptoms usually appear early in life, often between the ages of 3 and 6, and because symptoms vary from person to person, the disorder can be hard to diagnose. Parents may first notice that their child loses interest in things sooner than other children, or seems constantly "out of control." Often, teachers notice the symptoms first, when a child has trouble following rules, or frequently "spaces out" in the classroom or on the playground.

No single test can diagnose a child as having ADHD. Instead, a licensed health professional needs to gather information about the child, and his or her behavior and environment. A family may want to first talk with the child's pediatrician. Some pediatricians can assess the child themselves, but many will refer the family to a mental health specialist with experience in childhood mental disorders such as ADHD. The pediatrician or mental health specialist will first try to rule out other possibilities for the symptoms. For example, certain situations, events, or health conditions may cause temporary behaviors in a child that seem like ADHD. Between them, the referring pediatrician and specialist will determine if a child:

- Is experiencing undetected seizures that could be associated with other medical conditions
- Has a middle ear infection that is causing hearing problems
- Has any undetected hearing or vision problems
- Has any medical problems that affect thinking and behavior
- Has any learning disabilities
- Has anxiety or depression, or other psychiatric problems that might cause ADHD-like symptoms
- Has been affected by a significant and sudden change, such as the death of a family member, a divorce, or parent's job loss.

A specialist will also check school and medical records for clues, to see if the child's home or school settings appear unusually stressful or disrupted, and gather information from the child's parents and teachers. Coaches, babysitters, and other adults who know the child well also may be consulted. The specialist also will ask:

- Are the behaviors excessive and long-term, and do they affect all aspects of the child's life?
- Do they happen more often in this child compared with the child's peers?
- Are the behaviors a continuous problem or a response to a temporary situation?
- Do the behaviors occur in several settings or only in one place, such as the playground, classroom, or home?

The specialist pays close attention to the child's behavior during different situations. Some situations are highly structured, some have less structure. Others would require the child to keep paying attention. Most children with ADHD are better able to control their behaviors in situations where they are getting individual attention and when they are free to focus on enjoyable activities. These types of situations are less important in the assessment. A child also may be evaluated to see how he or she acts in social situations, and may be given tests of intellectual ability and academic achievement to see if he or she has a learning disability. Finally, if after gathering all this information the child meets the criteria for ADHD, he or she will be diagnosed with the disorder.

Chapter 5: Treatment of ADHD

How is ADHD treated?

Currently available treatments focus on reducing the symptoms of ADHD and improving functioning. Treatments include medication, various types of psychotherapy, education or training, or a combination of treatments.

Medications

The most common type of medication used for treating ADHD is called a "stimulant." Although it may seem unusual to treat ADHD with a medication considered a stimulant, it actually has a calming effect on children with ADHD. Many types of stimulant medications are available. A few other ADHD medications are non-stimulants and work differently than stimulants. For many children, ADHD medications reduce hyperactivity and impulsivity and improve their ability to focus, work, and learn. Medication also may improve physical coordination.

However, a one-size-fits-all approach does not apply for all children with ADHD. What works for one child might not work for another. One child might have side effects with a certain medication, while another child may not. Sometimes several different medications or dosages must be tried before finding one that works for a particular child. Any child taking medications must be monitored closely and carefully by caregivers and doctors.

Stimulant medications come in different forms, such as a pill, capsule, liquid, or skin patch. Some medications also come in short-acting, long-acting, or extended release varieties. In each of these varieties, the active ingredient is the same, but it is released differently in the body. Long-acting or extended release forms often allow a child to take the medication just once a day before school, so they don't have to make a daily trip to the school nurse for another dose. Parents and doctors should decide together which medication is best for the child and whether the child needs medication only for school hours or for evenings and weekends, too.

A list of medications and the approved age for use follows. ADHD can be diagnosed and medications prescribed by M.D.s (usually a psychiatrist) and in some states also by clinical psychologists, psychiatric nurse practitioners, and advanced psychiatric nurse specialists. Check with your state's licensing agency for specifics.

ADHD Medications Approved by U.S. Food and Drug Administration (FDA)*

Trade Name	Generic Name	Approved Age
Adderall	amphetamine	3 and older
Adderall XR	amphetamine (extended release)	6 and older
Concerta	methylphenidate (long acting)	6 and older
Daytrana	methylphenidate patch	6 and older
Desoxyn	methamphetamine hydrochloride	6 and older
Dexedrine	dextroamphetamine	3 and older
Dextrostat	dextroamphetamine	3 and older
Focalin	dexmethylphenidate	6 and older
Focalin XR	dexmethylphenidate (extended release)	6 and older
Metadate ER	methylphenidate (extended release)	6 and older
Metadate CD	methylphenidate (extended release)	6 and older
Methylin	methylphenidate (oral solution and chewable tablets)	6 and older
Ritalin	methylphenidate	6 and older
Ritalin SR	methylphenidate (extended release)	6 and older
Ritalin LA	methylphenidate (long acting)	6 and older
Strattera	atomoxetine	6 and older
Vyvanse	lisdexamfetamine dimesylate	6 and older

*Not all ADHD medications are approved for use in adults
NOTE: "extended release" means the medication is released gradually so that a controlled amount enters the body over a period of time. "Long acting" means the medication stays in the body for a long time.

Over time, this list will grow, as researchers continue to develop new medications for ADHD. Medication guides for each of these medications are available from the U.S. Food and Drug Administration (FDA) at www.fda.gov/cder/drug/infopage/ADHD/default.htm

What are the side effects of stimulant medications?
The most commonly reported side effects are decreased appetite, sleep problems, anxiety, and irritability. Some children also report mild stomachaches or headaches. Most side effects are minor and disappear over time or if the dosage level is lowered.

- Decreased Appetite: Be sure your child eats healthy meals. If this side effect does not go away, talk to your child's doctor. Also talk to the doctor if you have concerns about your child's growth or weight gain while he or she is taking this medication

- Sleep Problems: If a child cannot fall asleep, the doctor may prescribe a lower dose of the medication or a shorter-acting form. The doctor might also suggest giving the medication earlier in the day, or stopping the afternoon or evening dose. Adding a prescription for a low dose of an antidepressant or a blood pressure medication called clonidine sometimes helps with sleep problems. A consistent sleep routine that includes relaxing elements like warm milk, soft music, or quiet activities in dim light, may also help.

- Less Common Side Effects: A few children develop sudden, repetitive movements or sounds called tics. These tics may or may not be noticeable. Changing the medication dosage may make tics go away. Some children also may have a personality change, such as appearing "flat" or without emotion. **Talk with your child's doctor if you see any of these side effects.**

Are Stimulant Medications Safe?

Under medical supervision, stimulant medications are considered safe. Stimulants do not make children with ADHD feel high, although some kids report feeling slightly different or "funny." Although some parents worry that stimulant medications may lead to substance abuse or dependence, there is little evidence of this.

FDA Warning on Possible Rare Side Effects

In 2007, the FDA required that all makers of ADHD medications develop Patient Medication Guides that contain information about the risks associated with the medications. The guides must alert patients that the medications may lead to possible cardiovascular (heart and blood) or psychiatric problems. The agency undertook this precaution when a review of data found that ADHD patients with existing heart conditions had a slightly higher risk of strokes, heart attacks, and/or sudden death when taking the medications.

The review also found a slight increased risk, about 1 in 1,000, for medicationrelated psychiatric problems, such as hearing voices, having hallucinations, becoming suspicious for no reason, or becoming manic (an overly high mood), even in patients without a history of psychiatric problems. The FDA recommends that any treatment plan for ADHD include an initial health history, including family history, and examination for existing cardiovascular and psychiatric problems.

One ADHD medication, the non-stimulant atomoxetine (Strattera), carries another warning. Studies show that children and teenagers who take atomoxetine are more likely to have suicidal thoughts than children and teenagers with ADHD who do not take it. **If your child is taking atomoxetine, watch his or her behavior carefully. A child may develop serious symptoms suddenly, so it is important to pay attention to your child's behavior every day.** Ask other people who spend a lot of time with your child to tell you if they notice changes in your child's behavior. Call a doctor right away if your child shows any unusual behavior. While taking atomoxetine, your child should see a doctor often, especially at the beginning of treatment, and be sure that your child keeps all appointments with his or her doctor.

Do Medications Cure ADHD?
Current medications do not cure ADHD. Rather, they control the symptoms for as long as they are taken. Medications can help a child pay attention and complete schoolwork. It is not clear, however, whether medications can help children learn or improve their academic skills. Adding behavioral therapy, counseling, and practical support can help children with ADHD and their families to better cope with everyday problems. Research funded by the National Institute of Mental Health (NIMH) has shown that medication works best when treatment is regularly monitored by the prescribing doctor and the dose is adjusted based on the child's needs.

Psychotherapy
Different types of psychotherapy are used for ADHD. Behavioral therapy aims to help a child change his or her behavior. It might involve practical assistance, such as help organizing tasks or completing schoolwork, or working

through emotionally difficult events. Behavioral therapy also teaches a child how to monitor his or her own behavior. Learning to give oneself praise or rewards for acting in a desired way, such as controlling anger or thinking before acting, is another goal of behavioral therapy. Parents and teachers also can give positive or negative feedback for certain behaviors. In addition, clear rules, chore lists, and other structured routines can help a child control his or her behavior.

Therapists may teach children social skills, such as how to wait their turn, share toys, ask for help, or respond to teasing. Learning to read facial expressions and the tone of voice in others, and how to respond appropriately can also be part of social skills training.

How Can Parents Help?

Children with ADHD need guidance and understanding from their parents and teachers to reach their full potential and to succeed in school. Before a child is diagnosed, frustration, blame, and anger may have built up within a family. Parents and children may need special help to overcome bad feelings. Mental health professionals can educate parents about ADHD and how it impacts a family. They also will help the child and his or her parents develop new skills, attitudes, and ways of relating to each other.

Parenting skills training helps parents learn how to use a system of rewards and consequences to change a child's behavior. Parents are taught to give immediate and positive feedback for behaviors they want to encourage, and ignore or redirect behaviors they want to discourage. In some cases, the use of "time-outs" may be used when the child's behavior gets out of control. In a time-out, the child is removed from the upsetting situation and sits alone for a short time to calm down.

Parents are also encouraged to share a pleasant or relaxing activity with the child, to notice and point out what the child does well, and to praise the child's strengths and abilities. They may also learn to structure situations in more positive ways. For example, they may restrict the number of playmates to one or two, so that their child does not become overstimulated. Or, if the child has trouble completing tasks, parents can help their child divide large tasks into smaller, more manageable steps. Also, parents may benefit from learning stress-management techniques to increase their own ability to deal with frustration, so that they can respond calmly to their child's behavior.

Sometimes, the whole family may need therapy. Therapists can help family members find better ways to handle disruptive behaviors and to encourage behavior changes. Finally, support groups help parents and families connect with others who have similar problems and concerns. Groups often meet regularly to share frustrations and successes, to exchange information about recommended specialists and strategies, and to talk with experts.

Tips to Help Kids Stay Organized and Follow Directions

Schedule. Keep the same routine every day, from wake-up time to bedtime. Include time for homework, outdoor play, and indoor activities. Keep the schedule on the refrigerator or on a bulletin board in the kitchen. Write changes on the schedule as far in advance as possible.

Organize everyday items. Have a place for everything, and keep everything in its place. This includes clothing, backpacks, and toys.

Use homework and notebook organizers. Use organizers for school material and supplies. Stress to your child the importance of writing down assignments and bringing home the necessary books.

Be clear and consistent. Children with ADHD need consistent rules they can understand and follow.

Give praise or rewards when rules are followed. Children with ADHD often receive and expect criticism. Look for good behavior, and praise it.

Chapter 6: Coexisting Conditions with ADHD

What Conditions Can Coexist with ADHD?

Some children with ADHD also have other illnesses or conditions. For example, they may have one or more of the following:

- **A learning disability.** A child in preschool with a learning disability may have difficulty understanding certain sounds or words or have problems expressing himself or herself in words. A school-aged child may struggle with reading, spelling, writing, and math.

- **Oppositional defiant disorder.** Kids with this condition, in which a child is overly stubborn or rebellious, often argue with adults and refuse to obey rules.

- **Conduct disorder.** This condition includes behaviors in which the child may lie, steal, fight, or bully others. He or she may destroy property, break into homes, or carry or use weapons. These children or teens are also at a higher risk of using illegal substances. Kids with conduct disorder are at risk of getting into trouble at school or with the police.

- **Anxiety and depression.** Treating ADHD may help to decrease anxiety or some forms of depression.
- **Bipolar disorder.** Some children with ADHD may also have this condition in which extreme mood swings go from mania (an extremely high elevated mood) to depression in short periods of time.
- **Tourette syndrome.** Very few children have this brain disorder, but among those who do, many also have ADHD. Some people with Tourette syndrome have nervous tics and repetitive mannerisms, such as eye blinks, facial twitches, or grimacing. Others clear their throats, snort, or sniff frequently, or bark out words inappropriately. These behaviors can be controlled with medication.

ADHD also may coexist with a sleep disorder, bed-wetting, substance abuse, or other disorders or illnesses.

For more information on these disorders, visit www.nimh.nih.gov/health/topics/index.shtml

Recognizing ADHD symptoms and seeking help early will lead to better outcomes for both affected children and their families.

Chapter 7: Working With Your Child's School

How Can I Work with My Child's School?

If you think your child has ADHD, or a teacher raises concerns, you may be able to request that the school conduct an evaluation to determine whether he or she qualifies for special education services.

Start by speaking with your child's teacher, school counselor, or the school's student support team, to begin an evaluation. Also, each state has a Parent Training and Information Center and a Protection and Advocacy Agency that can help you get an evaluation. A team of professionals conducts the evaluation using a variety of tools and measures. It will look at all areas related to the child's disability

Once your child has been evaluated, he or she has several options, depending on the specific needs. If special education services are needed and your child is eligible under the Individuals with Disabilities Education Act, the school district must develop an "individualized education program" specifically for your child within 30 days.

If your child is considered not eligible for special education services—and not all children with ADHD are eligible—he or she still can get "free appropriate public education," available to all public-school children with disabilities under Section 504 of the Rehabilitation Act of 1973, regardless of the nature or severity of the disability.

The U.S. Department of Education's Office for Civil Rights enforces Section 504 in programs and activities that receive Federal education funds. For more information on Section 504, please see

www.ed.gov/about/offices/list/ocr/504faq.html

More information about Department of Education programs for children with disabilities is available at

www.ed.gov/parents/needs/speced/edpicks.jhtml?src=ln

Transitions can be difficult. Each school year brings a new teacher and new schoolwork, a change that can be especially hard for a child with ADHD who needs routine and structure. Consider telling the teachers that your child has ADHD when he or she starts school or moves to a new class. Additional support will help your child deal with the transition.

Chapter 8: Teens and ADHD

Do Teens with ADHD Have Special Needs?

Most children with ADHD continue to have symptoms as they enter adolescence. Some children, however, are not diagnosed with ADHD until they reach adolescence. This is more common among children with predominantly inattentive symptoms because they are not necessarily disruptive at home or in school. In these children, the disorder becomes more apparent as academic demands increase and responsibilities mount. For all teens, these years are challenging. But for teens with ADHD, these years may be especially difficult.

Although hyperactivity tends to decrease as a child ages, teens who continue to be hyperactive may feel restless and try to do too many things at once. They may choose tasks or activities that have a quick payoff, rather than those that take more effort, but provide bigger, delayed rewards. Teens with primarily attention deficits struggle with school and other activities in which they are expected to be more self-reliant. Teens also become more responsible for their own health decisions. When a child with ADHD is young, parents are more likely to be responsible for ensuring that their child maintains treatment. But when the child reaches adolescence, parents have less control, and those with ADHD may have difficulty sticking with treatment.

To help them stay healthy and provide needed structure, teens with ADHD should be given rules that are clear and easy to understand. Helping them stay focused and organized—such as posting a chart listing household chores and responsibilities with spaces to check off completed items—also may help.

Teens with or without ADHD want to be independent and try new things, and sometimes they will break rules. If your teen breaks rules, your response should be as calm and matter-offact as possible. Punishment should be used only rarely. Teens with ADHD often have trouble controlling their impulsivity and tempers can flare. Sometimes, a short time-out can be calming.

If your teen asks for later curfews and use of the car, listen to the request, give reasons for your opinions, and listen to your child's opinion. Rules should be clear once they are set, but communication, negotiation, and compromise are helpful along the way. Maintaining treatments, such as medication and behavioral or family therapy, also can help with managing your teenager's ADHD.

What About Teens and Driving?

Although many teens engage in risky behaviors, those with ADHD, especially untreated ADHD, are more likely to take more risks. In fact, in their first few years of driving, teens with ADHD are involved in nearly four times as many car accidents as those who do not have ADHD. They are also more likely to cause injury in accidents, and they get three times as many speeding tickets as their peers.

Most states now use a graduated licensing system, in which young drivers, both with and without ADHD, learn about progressively more challenging driving situations. The licensing system consists of three stages—learner's permit, during which a licensed adult must always be in the car with the driving teen; intermediate (provisional) license; and full licensure. Parents should make sure that their teens, especially those with ADHD, understand and follow the rules of the road. Repeated driving practice under adult supervision is especially important for teens with ADHD.

Chapter 9: Adults and ADHD

Can Adults have ADHD?

Some children with ADHD continue to have it as adults. And many adults who have the disorder don't know it. They may feel that it is impossible to get organized, stick to a job, or remember and keep appointments. Daily tasks such as getting up in the morning, preparing to leave the house for work, arriving at work on time, and being productive on the job can be especially challenging for adults with ADHD.

These adults may have a history of failure at school, problems at work, or difficult or failed relationships. Many have had multiple traffic accidents. Like teens, adults with ADHD may seem restless and may try to do several things at once, most of them unsuccessfully. They also tend to prefer "quick fixes," rather than taking the steps needed to achieve greater rewards.

How is ADHD Diagnosed in Adults?

Like children, adults who suspect they have ADHD should be evaluated by a licensed mental health professional. But the professional may need to consider a wider range of symptoms when assessing adults for ADHD because their symptoms tend to be more varied and possibly not as clear cut as symptoms seen in children.

To be diagnosed with the condition, an adult must have ADHD symptoms that began in childhood and continued throughout adulthood. Health professionals use certain rating scales to determine if an adult meets the diagnostic criteria for ADHD. The mental health professional also will look at the person's history of childhood behavior and school experiences, and will interview spouses or partners, parents, close friends, and other associates. The person will also undergo a physical exam and various psychological tests. For some adults, a diagnosis of ADHD can bring a sense of relief. Adults who have had the disorder since childhood, but who have not been diagnosed, may have developed negative feelings about themselves over the years. Receiving a diagnosis allows them to understand the reasons for their problems, and treatment will allow them to deal with their problems more effectively.

How is ADHD Treated in Adults?

Much like children with the disorder, adults with ADHD are treated with medication, psychotherapy, or a combination of treatments.

Medications

ADHD medications, including extended-release forms, often are prescribed for adults with ADHD, but not all of these medications are approved for adults. However, those not approved for adults still may be prescribed by a doctor on an "off-label" basis.

Although not FDA-approved specifically for the treatment of ADHD, antidepressants are sometimes used to treat adults with ADHD. Older antidepressants, called tricyclics, sometimes are used because they, like stimulants, affect the brain chemicals norepinephrine and dopamine. A newer antidepressant, venlafaxine (Effexor), also may be prescribed for its effect on the brain chemical norepinephrine. And in recent clinical trials, the antidepressant bupropion (Wellbutrin), which affects the brain chemical dopamine, showed benefits for adults with ADHD.

Adult prescriptions for stimulants and other medications require special considerations. For example, adults often require other medications for physical problems, such as diabetes or high blood pressure, or for anxiety and depression. Some of these medications may interact badly with stimulants. An adult with ADHD should discuss potential medication options with his or her doctor. These and other issues must be taken into account when a medication is prescribed.

Education and Psychotherapy
A professional counselor or therapist can help an adult with ADHD learn how to organize his or her life with tools such as a large calendar or date book, lists, reminder notes, and by assigning a special place for keys, bills, and paperwork. Large tasks can be broken down into more manageable, smaller steps so that completing each part of the task provides a sense of accomplishment.

Psychotherapy, including cognitive behavioral therapy, also can help change one's poor self-image by examining the experiences that produced it. The therapist encourages the adult with ADHD to adjust to the life changes that come with treatment, such as thinking before acting, or resisting the urge to take unnecessary risks.

Chapter 10: Research and Progress

What Efforts are Under Way to Improve Treatment?

This is an exciting time in ADHD research. The expansion of knowledge in genetics, brain imaging, and behavioral research is leading to a better understanding of the causes of the disorder, how to prevent it, and how to develop more effective treatments for all age groups.

NIMH has studied ADHD treatments for school-aged children in a large-scale, long-term study called the Multimodal Treatment Study of Children with ADHD (MTA study). NIMH also funded the Preschoolers with ADHD Treatment Study (PATS), which involved more than 300 preschoolers who had been diagnosed with ADHD. The study found that low doses of the stimulant methylphenidate are safe and effective for preschoolers, but the children are more sensitive to the side effects of the medication, including slower than average growth rates. Therefore, preschoolers should be closely monitored while taking ADHD medications.

PATS is also looking at the genes of the preschoolers, to see if specific genes affected how the children responded to methylphenidate. Future results may help scientists link variations in genes to differences in how people respond to ADHD medications. For now, the study provides valuable insights into ADHD.

Other NIMH-sponsored clinical trials on children and adults with ADHD are under way. In addition, NIMH-sponsored scientists continue to look for the biological basis of ADHD, and how differences in genes and brain structure and function may combine with life experiences to produce the disorder.

Other MedicalCenter.com Publications

The Key Facts on Arthritis

The Key Facts on Breast Cancer

The Key Facts on Medicare

The Key Facts on Cancer Types

The Key Facts on Cancer Treatment

The Key Facts on Cancer Risk Factors and
Causes

The Key Facts on Cancer Prevention

The Key Facts on Cancer Detection &
Diagnosis

The Key Facts on Coping With Cancer &
Cancer Resources

The Key Facts on Alzheimer's Disease

The Key Facts on Caring For Someone With
Alzheimer's Disease

The Key Facts on Obesity

The Key Facts on Diabetes

The Key Facts on Drug Abuse

All Titles Can Be Found at

www.Amazon.com

www.MedicalCenter.com

www.ingramcontent.com/pod-product-compliance
Lightning Source LLC
Chambersburg PA
CBHW070844290526
45795CB00002B/982